Marvelous
MEMORY
Boosters

Recharge Your Brain with Special Nutrients Proven to Boost Your Brain Power!

A Health Learning Handbook

Beth M. Ley, Ph.D.

BL Publications
Temecula, CA

BL Publications, Temecula, CA 92692 **877-BOOKS11**

Ley, Beth M. 1964-
    Marvelous Memory Boosters; Recharge Your Brain with Special Nutrients Proven to Boost Your Brain Power! /Beth M. Ley. 1st ed.
        p. cm. -- (A Health Learning Handbook)
    Includes bibliographical references and index.
    ISBN: 1-890766-09-7
    1. Nootropic agents 2. Dietary supplement. I. Title II. Series.

RM334.L49 1999
612.8'2--dc21   99-047612

Printed in the United States of America

First edition, January 2000

This book is not intended as medical advise. It's purpose is solely educational.

Credits:
Cover Design: Cuviello Graphic Design and BL Publications
Typesetting: BL Publications
Research and Technical Assistance: Keith Morey
Proofreading: Virginia Simpson-Magruder, Randi Nash

Table of Contents

The Brain: Our Memory Center

The brain, of course, is the control center of all physical and intellectual activity in the body. At birth the
human brain contains as many as one hundred billion
nerve cells. From then on there is a continuous process
of decline. Brain weight decreases gradually over time -
about 10% over a normal life span, due to neuron death.

Different parts of the brain lose neurons at different
rates. In most brain stem regions below the cerebral cortex (the area responsible for automatic unlearned activity (breathing, heart pumping, blinking, etc.), there is lit-
tle or no cell loss with advancing age. In comparison, the
cerebral cortex, which is responsible for thinking and
memory, loses up to 50,000 neurons a day.

The hippocampus is the specific region of the brain
known to be important for memory. New hippocampus
cells continually replace old one. Numerous factors determine the rate at which this is done. Factors which affect
overall mental functioning include:

- ✧ Optimal nutrition
- ✧ Oxidative stress (exposure to free radicals)
- ✧ Mental and physical stress (and other factors
  which effect cortisol (stress hormone) levels)
- ✧ Exposure to certain drugs (both recreational
  and pharmaceutical)
- ✧ Exposure to alcohol
- ✧ Environmental stimuli, (i.e. education)
- ✧ Genetics

More common than actual cell death is the loss of
the connections between neurons. With aging, dendritic
branching of the individual nerve cells decreases, reduc-
ing the number of connections between neurons.

Neuroscientists have long suspected that the

strength of the connections between neurons in the adult brain is susceptible to modification by ongoing neuronal activity. For example, if an adult rat is trained to run a complicated maze but its companion isn't, the maze-running rat will have a greater number of synapses. Other studies have confirmed that a greater amount of stimuli results in more learning and more synapses. If you want to expand your brain power, EXERCISE IT!

The losses of neurons and neuron synapses becomes more and more obvious as we get older. In some people, for reasons we are only beginning to learn about, this process is far more evident than others.

We are also just beginning to learn about the potential benefits of many nutrients - some new, some not.

The Nutrients:
For Enhanced Memory and Mental Function

The following nutrients have clinically demonstrated their importance in regards to memory, learning, concentration and other mental aspects, as well as treatment and prevention of mental related disorders such as senile dementia and Alzheimer's Disease.

Alpha-GPC (Alpha-Glycerylphosphorylcholine)

This is a derivative of soy lecithin that contains the essential nutrient choline. Alpha-GPC serves as a direct precursor in the synthesis of choline in the body. Choline, a part of the B Complex family, was recently acknowledged by the National Academy of Sciences as an essential nutrient by establishing an Adequate Intake (AI) level.

Choline is a precursor of the important neurotransmitter, acetylcholine. Choline supplementation increases the level of acetylcholine in the memory circuits of the temporal lobe of the brain. Acetylcholine-sensitive neurons serve many different functions in the brain including the control of arousal, learning, motor activity and deep sleep, known as Rapid Eye Movement (REM) sleep.

Studies conducted at the National Institutes of Health (NIH) showed that choline supplementation improves learning and memory in both normal individuals and in individuals with Alzheimer's. (Sitaram) It has also shown to enhance memory in young individuals.

In addition to its brain enhancing benefits, increased choline may also enhance Growth Hormone (GH) release. This effect may be even more pronounced in older individuals who may have depressed levels. GH levels significantly decline with age. The decline of GH is related to many symptoms of aging such as muscle atrophy, decreased energy and sexual function, increased body fat, increased risk of cardiovascular disease and osteoporosis, and wrinkles. Clinical evidence suggests that by replacing GH many of these symptoms can be reversed. Animal and human studies have demonstrated that Alpha-GPC stimulates the secretion of GH from the pituitary, making this supplement in high demand by all those concerned about aging! (Ghigo, Ceda)

Alpha-GPC may be useful to help reduce some of the neurological decline that occurs with aging as it has demonstrated significant beneficial effects upon cognitive function, memory impairments and dementia. (Frattola, Muratorio, Abbati, Di Perri)

Supplementing Alpha-GPC is preferred over supplementing choline or lecithin because Alpha-GPC allows for larger amounts of choline to be absorbed into the intestinal tract. (Zeisel)

Dosage: 100-500 mg. daily (Dosage may be reduced if taken in conjunction with other memory-enhancing nutrients.)

α–Lipoic Acid (Alpha Lipoic Acid)

α–Lipoic Acid is soluble in both water and fat. It is a powerful antioxidant that works synergistically with Vitamins C and E and glutathione, and helps regenerate C and E for re-use. It also supports the proper functioning of two key enzymes that convert food into energy.

The brain is subject to antioxidant stress just like the rest of the body. Antioxidant stress can contribute to circulatory problems and damage to brain cells. α–Lipoic Acid aids brain wellness because of its ability to neutralize potentially toxic substances and oxidants. (Siesjd, McCord)

The higher the level of antioxidants and the longer we can keep these antioxidants regenerating, the longer we are protected from oxidative damage. As antioxidant levels diminish, our vulnerability to neurological damage increases.

Animal studies have shown that α–Lipoic Acid is beneficial in helping to restore lost memory in aging subjects, but does not improve memory beyond what is normal in young healthy individuals. In mice, α–Lipoic Acid improved performance in an open-field memory test. The α–Lipoic Acid-treated animals actually performed slightly better than young animals 24 hours after the first test. The authors concluded that α–Lipoic Acid's free radical scavenging ability may improve N-methyl-o-aspartate receptor density, which leads to improved memory in older individuals. (Stoll)

α–Lipoic Acid also increases the energy availability in the brain in patients with a deficit of mitochondrial function. The mitochondria is the major energy-producing component in the cell.

Alzheimer's Disease is a neurodegenerative disorder characterized by loss of memory and progressive decline of cognitive abilities. Its cause is not entirely understood. The oxidative-stress hypothesis encourages antioxidant use for prevention and therapy. The toxicity of amyloid beta-protein, an amino acid peptide associated with plaques in the brains of Alzheimer's patients, seems also to be due to oxidative stress in neurons, and also potential sources of free radicals in brain tissue. (Behl)

Several other studies also suggest that free radicals are involved in the pathogenesis of Alzheimer's, and that antioxidant nutrients may be very useful in disease prevention. (Evans)

Parkinson's Disease is a brain disorder that causes muscle tremors, stiffness, and weakness. It is caused by degeneration to the basal ganglia in the brain nerve cells which may be caused by free radical damage.

A study based in the Netherlands suggested that a high intake of dietary antioxidants may protect against the occurrence of Parkinson's Disease. (de Rijk)

Researchers have proposed that inappropriate dopamine toxicity and or its oxidation products may initiate nigral cell loss in Parkinson's. Dopamine toxicity may be caused by the generation of free radicals. Neurology researchers in Israel found that the thiol family of antioxidants (glutathione, α–Lipoic Acid, etc.) is highly effective in rescuing cells from dopamine-induced death and may indeed be very beneficial for individuals with Parkinson's. (Offen)

Dosage: 50-400 mg. daily

Ascorbates (Vitamin C)

The brain is the second largest user of mineral ascorbates, the "true" form of Vitamin C, in the body. This should give you an idea of how important it is to help us think better and also to protect us, for example, to avoid stroke. Vitamin C is needed to produce many of the message carriers for the entire body, including serotonin, which is involved in regulation of appetite and sleep.

Mineral ascorbates (such as calcium or magnesium ascorbate) is the form of C that the body actually uses. Other forms of C, such as ascorbic acid, must first be converted into mineral ascorbates (calcium ascorbate, potassium ascorbates, etc,) in order to be used.

Antioxidants, such as ascorbate, which have been shown to reduce oxidative damage, may be protective against poor memory, which is a major component of dementia disorders such as Parkinson's and Alzheimer's.

Vitamin C levels are depressed among individuals with Alzheimer's, even though their intake of C-containing foods is similar to other individuals without Alzheimer's disease. (Riviere) At least one study has demonstrated the reduced incidence of Alzheimer's among individuals 65 years and older who supplement Vitamin C. (Morris)

Numerous studies suggest that Vitamin C protects against cognitive impairment. (Paleologos, Lonnrat) As a powerful antioxidant, ascorbate is protective of the neural tissues that are at risk of free radical damage.

Dosage: 2,000-8,000 mg. daily

Ashwagandha

This ancient Indian herb helps relieve stress, and is traditionally used for enhancement of memory, learning and sex drive. It promotes relaxation when sleep is desired by soothing the nerves and restoring strength. This herb may help reduce levels of elevated cortisol, which are associated with stress. Elevated cortisol levels are known to have a detrimental effect on memory by interfering with cell regeneration in the hippocampus region of the brain. (Suemaru, Newcomer)

It also has antioxidant properties, which may explain some of its pharmacological effects. (Panda)

Dosage: 100-200 mg. daily

B Complex Vitamins

B1 (Thiamine): This B Vitamin enhances circulation and assists in blood formation. It optimizes cognitive activity and brain function and has a positive effect on learning capacity and acts as an antioxidant. Thiamine plays a major role in the conversion of blood sugar into biological energy or "brain food."

 Dosage: 30-60 mg. daily

B2 (Riboflavin): B2 is necessary for red blood cell formation, antibody production, cell respiration and growth, as well as for the metabolism of tryptophan which is converted into niacin in the body. It aids in the metabolism of carbohydrates, fats and proteins, also alleviates eye fatigue.

 Dosage: 20-40 mg. daily

B3 (Niacin): Niacin, also known as nicotinic acid, is a vasodilator needed for proper circulation, and aids in the functioning of the nervous system. It is also a memory-enhancer. Niacin deficiency disease is known as pellagra. The early symptoms are fatigue, depression, and anxiety. Niacin-deficiency seems to be most responsible for rapid development of senility.

 Dosage: 15-20 mg. daily.

B5 (Pantothenic Acid): This nutrient is required for normal functioning of the nervous system. It is often called the "anti-stress" vitamin as it is involved in the production of neurotransmitters as well as adrenal hormones. B5 helps to convert fats, carbohydrates, and proteins into energy. It may provide nutritional support for recovery from depression and anxiety. B5 is required by the brain for conversion of choline into acetylcholine.

 Dosage: 100-500 mg. daily

B6 (Pyridoxine): This B Vitamin affects physical and mental health, is required by the nervous system, and is needed for normal brain function. It supports immune function and is needed to metabolize homocysteine to prevent plaque buildup in the arteries and arteriosclerosis.

Dosage: 20-40 mg. daily

B12 (Cyanocobalamin): B12 is linked to the production of acetylcholine, a neurotransmitter that assists in memory and learning. It helps prevent nerve damage and promotes normal growth and development. It is also important for the maintenance and protection of the fatty sheaths that cover and protect nerve endings.

Dosage: 15 mcg. daily

Folic Acid: Considered a brain food, Folic Acid is required for energy production and the formation of red blood cells. Folic Acid may also help depression and anxiety. Signs of deficiency include apathy, fatigue, insomnia, memory problems, anemia and labored breathing. Folic Acid is vital for fetal nerve development. Deficiencies of Folic Acid can cause low brain serotonin and depression. (Young)

Dosage: 800 mcg. daily

Bacopa Monniera

Bacopa monniera is an Ayurvedic botanical with apparent anti-anxiety, anti-fatigue, and memory-strengthening effects. It has been used historically for restoring cognitive function. (Kidd) It is well known as an adaptogen and a brain tonic for improving the intellect and increasing longevity.

Bacopa strengthens the veins and capillaries, thereby increasing circulation and delivery of oxygen and nutrients. Bacopa helps alleviate fatigue and promotes relaxation when sleep is desired. In addition to increasing brain function, concentration and memory, it may also increase sex drive.

There are also clinical trials demonstrating its anti-anxiety effect as it is one of the most popular supplements used in India for mental disorders and anxiety neurosis. (Singh, R.H.)

Dosage: 20 mg. daily

Boron

This important trace mineral enhances brain function, promotes alertness, and supports metabolism of calcium, phosphorus, and magnesium. The elderly benefit from supplementation as they have a greater problem with calcium absorption.

Studies show that boron deprivation results in decreased brain electrical activity. Assessments of cognitive and psychomotor function in humans found that boron deprivation results in poorer performance on tasks of motor speed and dexterity, attention, and short-term memory. (Penland)

Performance (e.g., response time) on various cognitive and psychomotor tasks also showed an effect of dietary boron. When contrasted with the high boron intake, low dietary boron resulted in significantly poorer performance on tasks emphasizing manual dexterity, eye-hand coordination, attention, perception, encoding and short-term memory, and long-term memory. (Penland, 1994)

Dosage: 2 mg. daily

CDP-Choline

CDP-Choline (Cytidine 5'-diphosphocholine), also known as Citicoline, is a source of choline involved in the biosynthesis of brain structural components (called phospholipids) and of acetylcholine (one of the major neurotransmitters in the brain). CDP-Choline is extensively used in the treatment of neurodegenerative diseases. Studies show CDP-Choline has vasoregulatory and neuroimmune actions and suggest that this compound may improve memory by acting on mechanisms of brain neurotropism and cerebrovascular regulation. (Alvarez)

CDP-Choline is an essential intermediate in the biosynthetic pathway of the lipid structural components of cell membranes, especially in that of phosphatidylcholine. Upon oral administration, it is absorbed almost completely, and its two principle components are released, cytidine and choline. Once absorbed, the cytidine and choline disperse widely throughout the body, cross the blood-brain barrier and reach the central nervous system (CNS), where they are incorporated into the membranes. CDP-Choline activates the biosynthesis of structural phospholipids in the neuronal membranes, increases cerebral metabolism, and acts on the levels of various neurotransmitters. It has been experimentally proven that CDP-Choline increases noradrenaline and dopamine levels in the CNS. Due to these pharmacological activities, CDP-Choline has a neuroprotective effect in situations of hypoxia and ischemia, as well as improved learning and memory performance in animal models of brain aging. (Secades)

Researchers investigated the effects of the oral administration of CDP-Choline (500-1,000 mg./day for 4 weeks) on memory performance in 24 elderly subjects with memory deficits and without dementia. Memory improved in free recall tasks, but not in recognition tests. A significant improvement in word recall, immediate object recall, and delayed object recall was observed after CDP-Choline treatment. A decrease in systolic blood pressure and minor changes in lymphocyte cell counting were also observed in elderly individuals after receiving CDP-Choline. (Alvarez)

CDP-choline was given to patients with Alzheimer's Disease at a daily dose of 1,000 mg./day for one month. Mental performance sightly increased, theta activity was reduced in fronto-temporal regions, increasing alpha power in occipital areas and cerebrovascular activity by increasing blood flow. (Cacabelos)

Dosage: 500-1,000 mg. daily. Dosages may be reduced if used in conjunction with other memory-enhancing nutrients.

CoQ10 (Coenzyme Q10)

The brain tissue contains a significant level of CoQ10 at 13.4 mcg. per gram. The prevalent existence of CoQ10 in the central nervous system suggests the potential usefulness of supplemental CoQ10 in the treatment of neuro-degenerative diseases.

The Proceeding of the National Academy of Sciences reports that CoQ10 supplementation, which increases brain mitochondrial concentrations, is neuroprotective.

In a study at Massachusetts General Hospital and Harvard Medical School, Boston, MA, oral administration of CoQ10 in 12-month-old rats resulted in significant increases in CoQ10 in the mitochondria in the cerebral cortex. It also markedly decreased damaged cells produced by administration of a known toxic substance. The CoQ10 also significantly increased the life span of the animals. (Matthews)

Individuals with Alzheimer's Disease have depressed CoQ10. (Edlund) While studies show that antioxidants such as Vitamin E are neuroprotective in individuals with

Alzheimer's, there are no published studies involving supplemental CoQ10 and this degenerative condition.

Researchers have also shown that CoQ10 levels are depressed in individuals with Parkinson's Disease. The energy-producing activities in platelet mitochondria are reduced in patients with early, untreated Parkinson's. CoQ10 is the electron acceptor for the energy-producing activities in the mitochondria. They found CoQ10 levels were significantly lower in mitochondria from Parkinson's patients and that CoQ10 levels and the mitochondrial activities were significantly correlated. (Shultz)

Researchers have reported that oral CoQ10 supplementation was beneficial in individuals with Parkinson's. Their pilot study examined the effects of 200 mg. CoQ10 administered two to four times per day for 1 month in 15 subjects with Parkinson's. While CoQ10 did not affect the motor portion of the Unified Parkinson's Disease Rating Scale, there was an increase in some mitochondrial activity. (Shultz)

Huntington's Disease is a rare, fatal, hereditary disorder resulting in death of brain cells. The symptoms are debilitating and include depression and loss of muscle coordination and cognitive function.

Studies also show that oral administration of CoQ10 significantly reduced increased concentrations of lactate, which suggests that CoQ10 might be useful in treating neurodegenerative diseases. (Beal)

Treatment with CoQ10 also significantly decreases cortical lactate concentrations in Huntington's patients, which reverses following withdrawal of therapy. These findings provide evidence for a generalized energy defect in Huntington's disease, and suggest a possible therapy with CoQ10. (Koroshetz)

Dosage: 200 mg. daily. High CoQ10 doses (600-1,200 mg. daily) have been used in some of the studies involving Parkinson's and Huntington's diseases to obtain beneficial results. These dosage levels were found to be safe and effective with only mild side effects. (Feigin)

DHA (Docosahexaenoic Acid)

DHA is an essential fatty acid (EFA), meaning it is an essential part of our daily diet. It is a member of the Omega-3 family, and is the longest of the long-chain polyunsaturated fatty acids (22:6n-3). It is the most sensitive to destruction and damage (mostly due to free radicals) both inside and outside the body. DHA is commonly deficient in the diet and body.

DHA: The Most Abundant Structural Fat in the Brain- DHA is of critical importance as it is the basic building block of each cell formed. Brain tissue is about 60% structural fat, of which about 25% is DHA. Brain and other nervous tissues are unique in containing this high concentration of DHA.

Each of the fourteen billion cells which make up the grey matter of the brain has connecting arms ending in synapses. These transport electrical currents between brain cells, sending messages throughout the body. When the arms are intact, communication is efficient. If the arms harden due to aging or free radical damage, signal transmission slows and may be altered. Adequate DHA helps keep the connections functional. Low levels can cause connections to lose efficiency, leading to brain and memory disorders.

Studies suggest that DHA supplementation may be helpful for the elderly, who require high levels of brain nutrients. Dr. Ernst Schaefer, of the Human Nutrition Center on Aging at Tufts University, reports that a low level of DHA is a significant risk factor for dementia- almost twice the risk of developing dementia over the next nine years than with those whose blood levels of DHA were high. (Schaefer)

In a Japanese study, patients taking 700-1,400 mg. DHA daily showed a large improvement in dementia symptoms (cooperation, speech, depression, and other psychological symptoms). The study found that the dementia in 69% of those individuals was due to blood vessel problems. (Yazawa)

The uptake of fatty acids into the neuronal tissue can be very slow and it may take six to eight months or longer to see changes in the brain and other nervous tissue. Many degenerative conditions do not develop "overnight" and cannot be expected to be reversed quickly either.

Alzheimer's Patients Have DHA Deficiency

Recent developments show that the brains of persons who have died from Alzheimer's Disease have an EFA deficiency, particularly DHA. Studies show that patients with Alzheimer's who receive EFA plus antioxidants show improvement consistently better than those not receiving fatty acids. (Corrigan)

Faulty brain cell membranes are also associated with the increased release of beta amyloid proteins. Beta amyloid proteins appear to be the principal active constituent of senile plaques thought to be a probable cause of brain damage resulting in Alzheimer's. (Newman)

DHA and other fatty acids are at high risk for oxidation in the brain, contributing to increased degradation of brain phospholipids in Alzheimer's disease. This was demonstrated by significantly decreased brain levels of membrane DHA and other fatty acids in Alzheimer's patients compared to control subjects. (Prasad)

This reinforces the importance of protective antioxidants which help prevent oxidative damage in the brain and throughout the body.

Dosage: 2,000-6,000 mg. (DHA/EPA combo) daily

DMAE

DMAE, short for Dimethylaminoethanol, is structurally very similar to choline, a nutrient necessary to make acetylcholine. Choline is involved in the process of learning and memory.

DMAE was given for four weeks to 14 outpatients to determine the safety of the supplement and whether it improves mental function. (Ferris) The dosage was gradually increased to 600 mg. three times daily during the first two weeks, with no adverse effects. Ten patients improved and four were unchanged. The patients on DMAE had reduced depression, irritability, and anxiety, as well as increased motivation. However, there were no apparent changes in memory.

DMAE users report that it stimulates thinking and motivation and increases the ability to focus better.

DMAE is potentially helpful for the elderly who have mental decline by improving alertness and focus. However, the long-term effectiveness of this nutrient is currently not known. DMAE is best reserved for occasional use on days when we have a special need to be more focused and alert. High dosages can cause irritability, anxiety, headaches, and neck and shoulder stiffness.

Dosage: 50-150 mg.

Ginkgo Biloba

Ginkgo biloba is powerful antioxidant herb that is best known for its ability to enhance circulation to the extremities (including the blood supply to the brain). It dilates the smallest capillaries to increase the supply of oxygen and nutrients, which aids in mental functioning. Research indicates that it may have some other, direct beneficial effects on mental performance, in addition to the effects of enhanced circulation and antioxidant protection.

With age, the blood flow in the brain decreases, which means less food and oxygen for brain cells. Reduced brain circulation can mean dizziness, memory loss, tinnitus (ringing in the ears), macular degeneration (the most common cause of blindness in the elderly), and even deafness (cochlear deafness). (Castleman)

Studies show that the components in Ginkgo help protect the sensitive brain cells from free radical molecules. (Eckmann) Ginkgo is known to pass through the blood brain barrier and therefore offer its protective benefits there as well as throughout the body. (Smith)

Numerous studies show that Ginkgo biloba extract helps us to maintain adequate antioxidant nutrition for our brain to function, such as remembering where you put your keys or glasses, what you were supposed to pick up at the grocery store or the directions to a place you haven't been in a few months. (Stoll, Grassel)

Dosage: 40 mg. daily (50:1-24%) Note: Higher amounts may cause headaches in some individuals.

Huperzine A

Huperzine A is a natural compound isolated from the Chinese botanical, club moss (Huperzia serrata), which has been used for centuries to improve memory, focus and concentration and to help alleviate memory problems among the elderly. It is safe with minimal side effects at therapeutic dosages.

Huperzine A is beneficial for brain functions as it is a potent and selective inhibitor of AChE (acetylcholinesterase), with a rapid absorption and penetration into the brain in experimental animals. The inhibition of AChE increases levels of acetylcholine.

Research has also demonstrated that Huperzine A protects nerve cells from toxins and from free radicals.

Huperzine A exhibits memory-enhancing activities in a broad range in animals. Researchers conclude that Huperzine A is a promising candidate for clinical development as a symptomatic treatment for Alzheimer's Disease. (Tang, Patocka) Huperzine A is safer than the drugs currently prescribed to Alzheimer's patients, but long term safety studies have not been done on normal individuals.

Dosage: 10-60 mcg. daily

L-Tyrosine

This amino acid is a precursor of norepinephrine and dopamine, which regulate or elevate mood. Supplementation may suppress the appetite, which may help to reduce body fat. It is also involved in the metabolism of phenylalanine. L-tyrosine may be useful for stress reduction, and research suggests it may be helpful as nutritional support to help the body cope with the effects of chronic fatigue, as well as anxiety, headaches, and the consequences of drug withdrawal.
Dosage: 150-500 mg. daily

Manganese

This trace mineral is needed for protein and fat metabolism, healthy nerves, healthy immune system, and blood sugar regulation. Manganese is used in energy production and works well with the B-complex vitamins to provide an overall feeling of well-being. Deficiency may cause confusion, memory loss, atherosclerosis, and eye and hearing problems.
Dosage: 15-50 mg. daily

MSM (Methyl-Sulfonyl-Methane)

MSM is a rich source of organic sulfur, the third largest occurring mineral in the body. It is a major detoxifier of the body, and is responsible for opening the sodium/potassium pump in every cell, allowing fluids and nutrients into the cell membrane while permitting toxins to exit. MSM is a great transporter for nutrients.
Dosage: 100 mg. to several grams daily

PS (Phosphatidylserine)

This nutrient is a naturally occurring phospholipid which is especially concentrated in the brain and nerve tissue. It is a critical component involved in brain function. Scientists believe that PS impacts the neuronal membranes and specific neurotransmitters such as acetylcholine, and studies show that PS may be able to diminish the negative effects of aging on cognitive ability.

The effects of PS have been validated through numerous double-blind trials for improving memory, learning, concentration, word recall, and mood in middle-aged and elderly subjects with dementia or age-related cognitive decline. PS is very safe.

In a study of 51 Alzheimer's patients, researchers gave 100 mg. of PS three times daily for 12 weeks. Those treated with PS showed improvement on several measures of cognitive function. (Crook)

PS is also known to reduce levels of elevated cortisol, which are associated with stress. (Monteleone) Elevated cortisol levels are detrimental to memory by interfering with cell regeneration in the hippocampus region of the brain. (Suemaru, Newcomer, Raber)

Another phospholipid, Phosphatidylcholine (PC), has also been studied extensively for its effects on intelligence and age-related loss of mental function, including Alzheimer's. Researchers at Massachusetts Institute of Technology (MIT), Cambridge, demonstrated that if there is inadequate dietary choline, the body will actually "steal" choline from its own neural membranes to produce acetylcholine. (Blusztajn) Some researchers speculate that this "mis-use" of choline, might explain some of the problems seen in Alzheimer's and other age-related memory disorders. (Maire)

PS and PC are not readily found in common foods. They are found in small amounts in lecithin (a component of egg yolks, wheat germ, and soy) and muscle meats.

Dosage: 100-200 mg. daily

Pregnenolone

Pregnenolone is a steriod hormone precursor. It is manufactured from cholesterol in the body and converts into progesterone, testosterone, estrogen, and DHEA. Unlike these other hormones, pregnenolone has powerful memory-enhancing effects (it also has no side effects compared to the others). In 1991 a rat study showed that pregnenolone was 100 time more effective at improving memory and learning tasks compared to other steriods. (Flood)

Studies indicate that pregnenolone reduces fatigue and stress, plays an important role in the acquisition of knowledge and long-term memory, and aiso promotes myelin formation during nerve regeneration.

Dosage: 50-300 mg. daily. When used with other memory enhancing nutrients, you may need to reduce the dosage.

TMG (Trimethylglycine)

TMG promotes healthy (controlled) levels of homocysteine, a toxic end product of the metabolism (methylation) of methionine, an essential amino acid. Homocysteine irritates the linings of veins and arteries, which researchers believe leads to cardiovascular deterioration. When methylation is working properly, homocysteine is quickly converted back to methionine, which is then converted to SAM (S-adenosylmethionine), a natural antidepressant. SAM then acts as a methyl donor for DNA, thereby protecting the DNA. SAM has also been shown to be useful in treating dementia and age-related depression, which may well be brought on by decreased methylation capacity resulting in lower levels of SAM.

Dosage: 100-200 mg. daily

Vinpocetine

This is a derivative of Vincamine, which is an extract of the common periwinkle plant (Vinca minor). It selectively dilates the arteries and capillaries in the head area, which improves circulation to the brain, thus alleviating cerebral insufficiency. Ongoing research around the world indicates that it may help improve memory, learning ability, insomnia, hearing, eyesight, and effects of menopause, and increase tolerance to damage caused by hypoxia (lack of oxygen, such as occurs with a stroke or heart attack).

Vinpocetine is often used for the treatment of cerebral circulatory disorders such as memory problems, acute stroke, aphasia (loss of the power of expression), apraxia (inability to coordinate movements), motor disorders, dizziness, and other cerebro-vestibular (inner-ear) problems, and headache. Vinpocetine is also used to treat acute or chronic ophthalmological diseases of various origin, with visual acuity improving in 70% of the subjects.

Gedeon Richter, a Hungarian company that markets Vinpocetine in Europe, has funded more than a hundred studies to show its effectiveness and safety. Many of these studies have shown the drug's powerful effect on memory improvement.

Vinpocetine is indeed a powerful memory enhancer. It facilitates cerebral metabolism by improving cerebral microcirculation (blood flow), stepping up brain cell ATP production (ATP is the cellular energy molecule), and utilization of glucose and oxygen.

What all this means is that Vinpocetine has a lot of the effects of several other cognitive enhancers all put together. Vinpocetine works great taken alone, and yet also works well when combined with other memory enhancing nutrients.

Vinpocetine improves four different and fundamental aspects of cerebral metabolism. Many studies have been performed on cerebral metabolism as it is immediate and practical to measure. But this is not the most interesting aspect of Vinpocetine. It is important to note that Vinpocetine is not only a cerebral vasodilator, but that its principal action, in a beneficial effect on the cerebral metabolism. In particular, the improvement of blood flow to the brain. (Kiss, Miyata)

4 ways Vinpocetine increases brain metabolism:

   1. It pumps up the blood flow.

   2. It increases the rate at which brain cells produce ATP (which is a cell molecule that creates energy).

   3. It speeds up the use of glucose in the brain.

   4. It speeds up the use of oxygen in the brain.

By acting in these four ways, vinpocetine improves overall cerebral efficiency resulting in brain cells that can better retain information–so the individual can remember more. Animal studies also show that Vinpocetine produces a significant and dose-dependent increase in the firing rate of neurons. The effective dose range was similar to the dose range corresponding to the memory-enhancing effects of the compound. This provides evidence that Vinpocetine increases the activity of ascending noradrenergic pathways – or in "English" – how fast the brain works. (Gaal)

Researchers have discovered that many degenerative brain disorders are accompanied by decreased circulation and diminished cellular efficiency. While the causes of common brain disorders are diverse and complex, it is reasonable to think that any agent which can enhance cerebral efficiency overall would thereby enhance cognitive function. This proves to be true in many cases with vinpocetine. Because of its stimulating effect on blood flow, Vinpocetine has been used to treat circulatory problems in the brain and memory problems due to low circulation.

Vinpocetine has been reported as showing promising

results in the treatment of tinnitus or ringing in the ears as well as other causes of impaired hearing. Vinpocetine has also been indicated in the treatment of strokes, menopausal symptoms and macular degeneration.

Literature suggests Vinpocetine may act to improve other conditions related to insufficient blood flow to the brain such as vertigo and Meniere's Syndrome, difficulty in sleeping, mood changes and depression.

It is important to remember that Vinpocetine has several different effects that have various important effects on cognitive function. The final result of the joint actions is the improvement of overall cognitive function.

While some Vinpocetine users notice cognitive improvements after a single dose or within the first few days, others may not see major improvement in medical situations for weeks or months. Improvements in cerebral disorders and in hearing and vision problems may last only as long as it is being taken on a regular basis.

Vinpocetine is safe for long term use. It is best to take Vinpocetine with food as mild and transient nausea, though rare, is more likely to occur when Vinpocetine is taken on an empty stomach.

Dosage: 10-40 mg. daily. Vinpocetine is normally taken orally, 5-10 mg., two or three times daily.

Vitamin E (Alpha-Tocopherol)

There is much written about the important antioxidant protective properties of alpha tocopherol.

Recently, Vitamin E has demonstrated its ability to prevent learning and memory deficits caused by amyloid beta-peptide, the major constituent of the senile plaques in the brains of patients with Alzheimer's. (Yamada)

Dosage: 600-1,200 IU daily

Zinc

This important mineral is required for protein synthesis and collagen formation. It promotes a healthy immune system and protects the liver from chemical damage. Deficiency may result in memory impairment, fatigue, high cholesterol levels, impaired night vision, weakened immune system, slow or impaired wound healing, and a propensity toward diabetes, prostate trouble, or impotence. Stress tends to deplete zinc stores from the body.

Studies have shown that depleted zinc levels are very common in Alzheimer's patients. (Corrigan)

Dosage: 10-25 mg. daily

Who Can Benefit from Memory Boosting Nutrients?

1. The elderly, as they have "severe" problems. But this is not necessarily the best user as cognitive deterioration is normally more advanced.

2. Anyone over 40. Cerebral arteriosclerosis is less well known to the public than heart disease, but it is just as common, and develops gradually over a lifetime. By the time serious symptoms develop, as with heart disease, the blood vessel occlusion is usually well advanced. Vinpocetine can minimize the structural, functional damage to brain neurons that may accompany gradually developing cerebral arteriosclerosis.

3. Baby boomers that are starting to suffer from symptoms of memory loss.

4. Young people, such as students, who want to enhance their memory - especially at examination time.

5. Anyone who has noticed a decrease in memory, alertness, concentration, learning speed ability, neuro-muscular co-ordination and reaction time, vision, hearing, or who suffers from tinnitus.

6. Anyone who suffers from, or is known to be at risk for, various cerebral disorders, cerebral hemorrhage, stroke, senile dementia, transient ischaemic attacks, chronic cerebral circulatory insufficiency, etc.

7. Anyone who has abused various brain toxic substances in the past. These include:
  - ✧ Alcohol, opiates (morphine, heroine), cocaine, amphetamines and hallucinogens (STP, MDA, marijuana, LSD, etc.) and barbiturates.

8. Anyone who had used various prescribed psychiatric drugs which may be very toxic to the brain causing memory loss, confusion or depression. These include:
  - ✧ Pain killers, antidepressants, sleeping pills and tranquilizers such as Valium (diazepam) and Ativan, Thoazine, Stelazine, Haldol and lithium.

Other medications that may have an adverse effect on brain function include:
  - ✧ Antihistimines, often taken for allergies.

  - ✧ Corticosteriods, antiinflammatory agents pre scribed for a variety of reasons such as asthma, arthritis, etc.

  - ✧ Heart and blood pressure medication such as digitalis, Inderal and reserpine.

  - ✧ Anti-asthma medications such as aminophylline.

  - ✧ Anti-gastric drugs, such as cimetidine.

Combining too many different medications can also be very toxic to the brain.

Bibliography

Abbiati, G., et al; Nootropic therapy of cerebral aging. Advances in therapy, Vol. 8, No. 6, 1991;268-276.

Alvarez XA; Laredo M; Corzo D; Fernandez-Novoa L; Mouzo R;Perea JE; Daniele D; Cacabelos R Citicoline improves memory performance in elderly subjects. Methods Find Exp Clin Pharmacol 1997 Apr;19(3):201-10.

Barbiroli, B., Medori, R., Tritschler, H.J., et al: Lipoic (thioctic) acid increases brain energy availability and skeletal muscle performance as shown by in vivo 31P-MRS in a patient with mitochondrial cytopathy. J Neurol 1995 Jul;242(7):472-7.

Beal MF; Matthews RT; Coenzyme Q10 in the central nervous system and its potential usefulness in the treatment of neurodegenerative diseases. Massachusetts General Hospital, Boston Mol Aspects Med 1997; 18 Suppl:S169-7960.

Beal, MF, et al; Coenzyme Q10 and nicotinamide block striatal lesions produced by the mitochondrial toxin malonate, Annals of Neurology, 1994;36;882-8.

Behl C, Amyloid beta-protein toxicity and oxidative stress in Alzheimer's disease. Max Planck Institute of Psychiatry, Clinical Institute, Kraepelinstr. 2-10, D-80804 Munich, Germany. chris@mpipsykl.mpg.de Cell Tissue Res 1997 Dec;290(3):471-80

Behl C; Sagara YMechanism of amyloid beta protein induced neuronal cell death: current concepts and future perspectives. J Neural Transm Suppl 1997;49:125-34

Bhatti JZ; Hindmarch I; Vinpocetine effects on cognitive impairments produced by fluni-trazepam. Int Clin Psychopharmacol 1987 Oct;2(4):325-31.

Blusztajn JK; Liscovitch M; Mauron C; et al; Phosphatidylcholine as a precursor of choline for acetylcholine synthesis. Neural Transm Suppl 1987;24:247-59.

Cameron HA; McKay R; Stem cells and neurogenesis in the adult brain. Laboratory of Molecular Biology, National Institutes of Health, Bethesda, Maryland Curr Opin Neurobiol 1998 Oct;8(5):677-80.

Cacabelos R; Caamano J; et al; Therapeutic effects of CDP-choline in Alzheimer's disease. Cognition, brain mapping, cerebrovascular hemodynamics, and immune factors. Institute for CNS Disorders, Basic and Clinical Neurosciences Research Center, La Coruna, Spain, Ann N Y Acad Sci 1996 Jan 17;777:399-403.

Ceda, G.P., et al; Effects pfCytidine5'Diphosphocholine administration on basal and GH releaseing secretion in elderly subjects, Acta Endocrinol. 1991. May; 124(5) 516-520.

Ceda, G.P., et al.; Alpha-GPC administration increases GH responses to GHRH of young and elderly sunjects. Horm. Metab. Res. 1992 Mar;24(3):119-121.

Corrigan FM; Van Rhijn AG; Horrobin, DF.; EFAs in Alxheimer's Disease. Ann NY AcadAci , 1991;6640:250-2.

Corrigan FM; Reynolds GP; Ward NI; Hippocampal tin, aluminum and zinc in Alzheimer's disease. Argyll & Bute Hospital, Lochgilphead, UK. Biometals 1993 Autumn;6(3):149-54.

Corrigan FM; Mowat B; et al.; High density lipoprotein fatty acids in dementia. Argyll and Bute NHS Trust, Argyll and Bute Hospital, Lochgilphead, UK. Prostaglandins Leukot Essential Fatty Acids 1998 Feb;58(2):125-7.

Crook, T., et al; Effects of phosphatidlyserine in Alzheimer's disease. Psychopharmacol Bull. 1992;28:61-6.

Edlund C; et al Ubiquinone, dolichol, and cholesterol metabolism in aging and Alzheimer's disease. Biochem Cell Biol 1992 Jun;70(6):422-8.

Eriksson PS; Perfilieva E; Bjork-Eriksson T; Alborn AM; Nordborg C; Peterson DA;Neurogenesis in the adult human hippocampus. Nat Med 1998 Nov;4(11):1313-7.

Erdo SA; Molnar P; Lakics V; Bence JZ; Tomoskozi Z; Vincamine and vincanol are potent blockers of voltage-gated Na+ channels. Laboratory of CNS Pharmacology, Chinoin Co., Budapest, Hungary. Eur J Pharmacol 1996 Oct 24;314(1-2):69-73.

Evans DA; Morris MC, Is a randomized trial of antioxidants in the primary prevention of Alzheimer disease warranted? Alzheimer Dis Assoc Disord 1996 Fall;10 Suppl 1:45-9.

Ferris, S.H., et al. "Senile dementia: treatment with deanol," J. Ant. Geriatr. Soc. 25(6):241-4, 1977.

Flood, JF, Morley, JE et al.: Memory enhancing effects in male rats of pregnenolone and ste-riods metabolically derived from it. Proc Natl Acad Sci 89:1567-71, March 92.

Gaal L; Molnar P; Effect of vinpocetine on noradrenergic neurons in rat locus coeruleus. Eur J Pharmacol 1990 Oct 23;187(3):537-9.

Ghigo, E, et al; Loe doses of either IV or orally administered arginine are able to enhance GH response to GHRHsecretion in elderly subjects, J. Endocrinol Invest. 1994, Feb;17(2):113-117.

Gotz ME, Dirr A, Gsell W, Burger R, Janetzky B, Freyberger A, Reichmann H, Rausch WD, Riederer P Influence of N-methyl-4-phenyl-1,2,3,6-tetrahydropyridine, a-Lipoic Acid and L-deprenyl on the interplay between cellular redox systems. J Neural Transm Suppl

1994;43:145-62.

Grassel E Effect of Ginkgo-biloba extract on mental performance. Double-blind study using computerized measurement conditions in patients with cerebral insufficiency Fortschr Med 1992 Feb 20;110(5):73-6

Kidd PM; A review of nutrients and botanicals in the integrative management of cognitive dysfunction Contributing Editor, Alternative Medicine Review. Correspondence address:47 Elm St., El Cerrito, CA. Altern Med Rev 1999 Jun;4(3):144-61.

Kiss B; Karpati E; [Mechanism of action of vinpocetine] Vinpocetin hatasai, hatasmechanizmusa. Richter Gedeon Vegyeszeti Gyar Rt., Farmakologiai Kutato Kozpont, Budapest.Acta Pharm Hung 1996 Sep;66(5):213-24.

Koroshetz WJ; Jenkins BG; Rosen BR; Beal MF; Energy metabolism defects in Huntington's disease and effects of coenzyme Q10. Neurology Service, Mass. General Hospital and Harvard Medical School, Boston. Ann Neurol 1997; Feb;41(2):160-546.

Lakics V; Sebestyen MG; Erdo SL;Vinpocetine is a highly potent neuroprotectant against veratridine- induced cell death in primary cultures of rat cerebral cortex. CNS Pharmacology Lab, Budapest, Hungary. Neurosci Lett 1995 Feb 9;185(2):127-30.

Lonnrot K; Metsa-Ketela T; et al; *The effect of ascorbate and ubiquinone supplementation on plasma and CSF total antioxidant capacity.* Free Radic Biol Med 1996;21(2):211-7.

Maire JC; Wurtman RJ; Choline production from choline-containing phospholipids: a hypothetical role in Alzheimer's disease and aging. Prog Neuropsycho-pharmacol Biol Psychiatry 1984;8(4-6):637-42.

Miyazaki M; The effect of a cerebral vasodilator, vinpocetine, on cerebral vascular resistance evaluated by the Doppler ultrasonic technique in patients with cerebrovascular diseases. Department of Internal Medicine, Rohju Sanatorium, Osaka, Japan.Angiology 1995 Jan;46(1):53-8.

Miyata N; Yamaura H; Tanaka M; et al; Effects of VA-045, a novel apovincaminic acid derivative, on isolated blood vessels: cerebroarterial selectivity. Research Center, Taisho Pharmaceutical Co., Ltd., Saitama, Japan. Life Science

Monteleone P; Maj M; Beinat L; Natale M; Kemali DBlunting by chronic phosphatidylserine administration of the stress- induced activation of the hypothalamo-pituitary-adrenal axis in healthy men. Institute of Psychiatry, First Medical School, University of Naples, Italy. Eur J Clin Pharmacol 1992;42(4):385-8.

Monteleone P; Beinat L; Tanzillo C; Maj M; Kemali D Effects of phosphatidylserine on the neuroendocrine response to physical stress in humans. Institute of Medical Psychology and Psychiatry, First Medical School, University of Naples, Italy. Neuroendocrinology 1990 Sep;52(3):243-8.

Morris, MC; et al; Vitamin E and Vitamin C Supplement Use and Risk of Incident Alzheimer Disease, Alzheimer Disease and Associated Disorders; Vol 112; No 3, 121-126.

Newcomer JW; Selke G; Melson AK; et al;Decreased memory performance in healthy humans induced by stress-level cortisol treatment. Department of Psychiatry, Washington University School of Medicine, St Louis, MO. Arch Gen Psychiatry 1999 Jun;56(6):527-33.

Newman PE; Could diet be one of the causal factors of Alzheimer's disease? Source: Med Hypotheses, 1992 Oct, 39:2, 123-6.

Nilsson M; Perfilieva E; Johansson U; Orwar O; Eriksson PS; Enriched environment increases neurogenesis in the adult rat dentate gyrus and improves spatial memory. J Neurobiol 1999 Jun 15;39(4):569-78.

Nosalova V; Machova J; Babulova A; Protective action of vinpocetine against experimentally induced gastric damage in rats. Institute of Experimental Pharmacology, Slovak Academy of Sciences, Bratislava.Arzneimittelforschung 1993 Sep;43(9):981-5.

Offen D; Ziv I; Sternin H; Melamed E; Hochman A Prevention of dopamine-induced cell death by thiol antioxidants: possible implications for treatment of Parkinson's disease. Exp Neurol 1996 Sep;141(1):32-9

Okuyama S; Hashimoto-Kitsukawa S; Ogawa S; Imagawa Y; et al; Effects of VA-045, a novel apovincaminic acid derivative, on age- related impairment evidence in electroencephalograph, caudate spindle, a passive avoidance task and cerebral blood flow in rats. Gen Pharmacol 1994 Nov;25(7): 1311-20

Orvisky E; Soltes L; Stancikova M; High-molecular-weight hyaluronan—a valuable tool in testing the antioxidative activity of amphiphilic drugs stobadine and vinpocetine. J Pharm Biomed Anal 1997 Nov;16(3):419-24.

Paleologos M; Cumming RG; et al; *Cohort study of vitamin C intake and cognitive impairment.* University of Sydney, New South Wales, Australia.Am J Epidemiol 1998 Jul 1;148(1):45-50.

Panda S; Kar A Evidence for free radical scavenging activity of Ashwagandha root powder in mice. Indian J Physiol Pharmacol 1997 Oct;41(4):424-6.

Patocka J; Huperzine A--an interesting anticholinesterase compound from the Chinese herbal medicine. Acta Medica (Hradec Kralove) 1998;41(4):155-7.

Penland JG; The importance of boron nutrition for brain and psychological function. US Depart of Agriculture. Biol Trace Elem Res 1998 Winter;66(1-3):299-317.

Penland JG; Dietary boron, brain function, and cognitive performance. US Department of Agriculture, Environ Health Perspect 1994 Nov;102 Suppl 7:65-72.

Prasad MR; Markesbery WR; Dhillon H; Yatin MLovell MA Regional membrane phospholipid alterations in Alzheimer's disease. Department of Surgery, University of Kentucky, Lexington Neurochem Res 1998 Jan;23(1):81-8.

Pudleiner P; Vereczkey L; Study on the absorption of vinpocetine and apovincaminic acid. Chemical Works of Gedeon Richter Ltd, Budapest, Hungary. Eur J Drug Metab Pharmacokinet 1993 Oct-Dec;18(4):317-21.

Raber J; Detrimental effects of chronic hypothalamic-pituitary-adrenal axis activation. From obesity to memory deficits. 94141-9100, USA. Mol Neurobiol 1998 Aug;18(1):1-22.

Riviere S; Birlouez-Aragon I; Nourhashemi F; Vellas B; Low plasma vitamin C in Alzheimer patients despite an adequate diet. Int J Geriatr Psychiatry 1998 Nov;13(11):749-54

Secades JJ; Frontera G; CDP-choline: pharmacological and clinical review. Methods Find Exp Clin Pharmacol 1995 Oct;17 Suppl B:2-54.

Shults CW; Haas, RH; Beal, MF; A Possible Role of Coenzyme Q10 in the etiology and treatment of Parkinson's Disease,University of Cafifornia, San Diego, La Jolla, Neurology Service, VA Health Care System, San Diego, Massachusetts General Hospital, Boston.

Singh RB; Treatment.Standard plus Q gel 2caps twice daily showing relief. J of Nutr and Environ Med,UK,1999.

Singh RB; Niaz MA; Rastogi SS; et al; Effect of hydrosoluble coenzyme Q10 on blood pressures and insulin resistance in hypertensive patients with coronary artery disease. J Hum Hypertens 1999 Mar;13(3):203-8.

Singh RB; Wander GS; Rastogi A; et al; Randomized, double-blind placebo-controlled trial of coenzyme Q10 in patients with acute myocardial infarction. Cardiovasc Drugs Ther 1998 Sep;12(4):347-53.

Singh RH; Studies on the Anti-anxiety effect of the Medhya Rasayana Drug (Bacopa Monniera) Department of Kayacikitsa, Institue of Medical Sciences, Banara Hindu University, Varansi-5, India, January 1978.

Sopher BL; Martin GM; Furlong CE; Kavanagh TJ; Neurodegenerative mechanisms in Alzheimer disease. A role for oxidative damage in amyloid beta protein precursor-mediated cell death. Mol Chem Neuropathol 1996 Oct-Dec;29(2-3):153-68

Subhan Z; Hindmarch I; Psychopharmacological effects of vinpocetine in normal healthy volunteers. Eur J Clin Pharmacol 1985;28(5):567-71.

Suemaru S; et al; J Cerebrospinal fluid corticotropin-releasing hormone and ACTH, and peripherally circulating choline-containing phospholipid in senile dementia. Life Sci 1993;53(9):697-706.

Stoll, S., Hartmann, H., et al The potent rree radical scavanger a-Lipoic Acid improved memory in aged mice. Putative relationship to NMDA receptor deficits. Pharmacol. Biochem. Behav (1993) 36:799-805.

Stoll S; Scheuer K; Pohl O; Muller WE Ginkgo biloba extract (EGb 761) independently improves changes in passive avoidance learning and brain membrane fluidity in the aging mouse. Pharmacopsychiatry 1996 Jul;29(4):144-9

Szakall S; Boros I; Balkay L; Emri M; Fekete I; Kerenyi L; Lehel S; Marian T; Molnar T; Varga J; Galuska L; Tron L; Bereczki D; Csiba L; Gulyas B;Cerebral effects of a single dose of intravenous vinpocetine in chronic stroke patients: a PET study. Debrecen University Medical School, Hungary. J Neuroimaging 1998 Oct;8(4):197-204.

Tang XCHuperzine A (shuangyiping): a promising drug for Alzheimer's disease, State Key Lab of Drug Research, Shanghai Institute of Materia Medica, Chinese Academy of Sciences, China. Chung Kuo Yao Li Hsueh Pao 1996 Nov;17(6):481-4.

Tohgi H; Sasaki K; Chiba K; Effect of vinpocetine on oxygen release of hemoglobin and erythrocyte organic polyphosphate concentrations in patients with vascular dementia of the Binswanger type.Arzneimittelforschung 1990 Jun;40(6):640-3.

Wei Y; Shi NC; et al; J Inhibitory effects of vinpocetine on sodium current in rat cardiomyocytes.Chung Kuo Yao Li Hsueh Pao 1997 Sep;18(5):411-5.

Yamada K; Tanaka T; Han D; Senzaki K; Kameyama T; Protective effects of idebenone and alpha-tocopherol on beta-amyloid-(1- 42)-induced learning and memory deficits in rats: implication of oxidative stress in beta-amyloid-induced neurotocity in vivo. Eur J Neurosci 1999 Jan;11(1):83-90.

Yazawa, K.; Clinical esperience with DHA in demented patients. International Conference on Highly Unsaturatd Fatty Acids in Nutritio and Desise Prevention. Barcelone. Spain. 1996. November 4-6.

Young SN; The 1989 Borden Award Lecture. Some effects of dietary components (amino acids, carbohydrate, folic acid) on brain serotonin synthesis, mood, and behavior. Can J Physiol Pharmacol 1991 Jul;69(7):893-903.

Zeisel, S. et al.; Dietary Choline: Biochemistry, Physioogy and Pharmacology. Ann. Rev. Nutr. 1981. 1:95-121.

Index

YOU NEED TO KNOW...
THE HEALTH MESSAGE

BOOKS AVAILABLE FROM BL PUBLICATIONS:

Send book order total amount plus $2 shipping by check or money order to: BL Publications, 39341 San Thomas Ct. Murrieta, CA 92562. Credit card orders: **1-877-BOOKS11**

A Diet For The Mind by Fred Chapur, 112 pages $8.95

Aspirin Alternatives: The Top Natural Pain-Relieving Analgesics
by Raymond Lombardi, D.C., C.C.N., 160 pages $8.95

Castor Oil: Its Healing Properties by Beth M. Ley, 36 pages $3.95

Dr. John Willard on Catalyst Altered Water by Beth M. Ley, 60 pages . . . $3.95

Coenzyme Q10: All-Around Nutrient for All-Around Health
by Beth M. Ley Jacobs, Ph.D., 70 pages $4.95

Colostrum: Nature's Gift to the Immune System by Beth M. Ley, 80 pages . $4.95

DHA: The Magnificent Marine Oil by Beth Ley Jacobs, Ph.D., 120 pages . .$6.95

DHEA: Unlocking the Secrets of the Fountain of Youth- Second Edition
by Beth M. Ley and Richard Ash, M.D., 256 pages $14.95

Health Benefits of Probiotics
by Dr. S.K. Dash, Dr. Allan Spreen, 56 pages $4.95

How Did We Get So Fat?
by Arnold J. Susser, R.P. Ph.D., & Beth M. Ley, 96 pages $7.95

How to Fight Osteoporosis and Win! The Miracle of Microcrystalline
Hydroxyapatite by Beth M. Ley, 80 pages $6.95

Marvelous Memory Boosters by Beth M. Ley, Ph.D., 32 pages $3.95

MSM: On Our Way Back to Health With Sulfur by Beth M. Ley, 40 pages $3.95

Natural Healing Handbook
by Beth M. Ley w/ foreword by Arnold J. Susser, R.P., Ph.D., 320 pages . $14.95

Nature's Road to Recovery: Nutritional Supplements for the Alcoholic and
Chemical Dependent by Beth M. Ley Jacobs, Ph.D., 72 pages $5.95

PhytoNutrients: Medicinal Nutrients Found in Foods
by Beth M. Ley, 40 pages $3.95

The Potato Antioxidant: Alpha Lipoic Acid by Beth M. Ley, 96 pages . . . $6.95

Vinpocetine: Revitalize Your Brain with Periwinkle Extract!
by Beth M. Ley, Ph.D., 48 pages $4.95